URINARY TRACT INFECTION (UTI) RECIPES FOR NEWLY DIAGNOSED

Discover Nutritional Solutions, Proven Strategies, Meal Plans, Medical Insights, And Lifestyle Tips To Combat UTIs And Promote Healthy Living

DR. ERIC TRISTAN

CONTENTS

DISCLAIMER

The information provided in this book, is intended for informational purposes only. The content is not intended to be a substitute for professional medical advice, diagnosis, or treatment. Always seek the advice of your physician or other qualified health provider with any questions you may have regarding a medical condition. Never disregard professional medical advice or delay in seeking it because of something you have read in this book.

The author of this book has made reasonable efforts to ensure that the information provided is accurate and up-to-date at the time of publication. However, the author makes no representations or warranties of any kind, express or implied, about the completeness, accuracy, reliability, suitability, or availability of the information contained within these pages.

Any reliance you place on the information provided in this book is strictly at your own risk. The author shall not be liable for any loss, injury, or damage arising from the use of this book or the information contained herein.

The mention or reference to any individuals, products, websites, organizations, or other names within this book does not imply endorsement by the author. The inclusion of such references is solely for informational purposes and does not constitute an endorsement or recommendation.

Furthermore, the author disclaims any association or affiliation with any individuals, products, websites, organizations, or other names mentioned in this book.

It is important to consult with a qualified healthcare professional before making any dietary or lifestyle changes, especially if you have a medical condition. Each individual's health situation is unique, and what works for one person may not work for another.

Again, the information provided in this book is not intended to diagnose, treat, cure, or prevent any disease or health condition. Always seek the advice of a physician or other qualified health provider regarding any medical questions or concerns you may have.

Thank you for your understanding and for taking the necessary precautions when considering the information presented in this book.

ABOUT THIS BOOK

This book titled "Urinary Tract Infection (UTI) Recipes" provides an all-encompassing manual that aids readers in their efforts to comprehend, avert, and control urinary tract infections (UTIs). The introduction establishes the framework for the following chapters and provides context for the significance of addressing urinary tract infections. "Understanding Urinary Tract Infections (UTIs)" provides a comprehensive analysis of UTIs, elucidating their etiology and risk factors; thus, it equips readers with essential information for proactive prevention.

The subsequent segments, "Symptoms and Diagnosis" and "Prevention Strategies," provide readers with the necessary knowledge to accurately identify and effectively manage urinary tract infections (UTIs). By emphasizing the importance of hydration in UTI prevention, this book demonstrates its dedication to providing practical guidance. With evidence-based insights, a chapter devoted to the correlation between cranberry and urinary tract infections (UTIs) investigates a remedy that is extensively debated.

By integrating dietary solutions, "Probiotics for UTI Prevention" further broadens the scope of preventive measures. This book provides a systematic delineation of "Foods to Incorporate into a UTI-Friendly Diet" and "UTI-Friendly Beverages," offering a methodical framework for selecting beverages and foods that promote urinary health.

In "Recipes for UTI Relief," this book provides concrete remedies that surpass broad principles, appealing to individuals who are actively engaged in the management of UTIs. This book "Herbal Teas for UTI Support" and "UTI-Friendly Snack Ideas" offer delectable substitutes, thereby enhancing the variety and palatability of the voyage toward managing UTIs. The inclusion of "Nutritional Supplements for UTI Prevention" enhances the book's dedication to comprehensive health.

Acknowledging the significance of expert counsel, the incorporation of "Consulting a Healthcare Professional" in the text encourages readers to pursue individualized recommendations. In summary, this book serves as an indispensable resource, facilitating the transition from knowledge of urinary tract infections to the adoption of health-conscious, practicable lifestyle modifications required for efficient management.

CHAPTER ONE

An Overview Of Recipes For Urinary Tract Infections (UTIS)

Regardless of gender or age, urinary tract infections (UTIs) are a prevalent and frequently distressing health condition that can impact any individual. Although medical intervention is essential for the treatment of urinary tract infections (UTIs), integrating specific recipes into one's dietary regimen may promote urinary tract health and potentially avert recurrent infections. This article will discuss the significance of diet in the management of urinary tract infections (UTIs) and offer recipes that can be used in conjunction with medical treatments.

A Comprehension Of Urinary Tract Infections

It is vital to have a thorough understanding of what a UTI is and how it develops before discussing recipes. Undertakings (UTIs) are caused by the entry and multiplication of bacteria, usually Escherichia coli (E. coli), which subsequently develop into an infection. The ureters, urethra, kidneys, and bladder comprise the urinary tract. UTIs are more prevalent in women because their urethras are shorter, which facilitates bacterial entry into the bladder.

Diverse urinary tract infections (UTIs) may result from the infection, including cystitis (infection of the bladder), pyelonephritis (infection of the kidneys), and urethritis (infection of the urethra). Urinary tract infections (UTIs) may result in urinary distress and pain, frequent urinary urgency, and lower abdominal pain. A comprehensive knowledge of the physiology and anatomy of the urinary tract is essential for effective prevention and treatment.

Risk Factors And Etiology Of Urinary Tract Infections

Multiple contributing factors contribute to the onset of urinary tract infections (UTIs). The ingress of bacteria into the urinary tract is the principal etiology. This can occur via the urethra, frequently as a result of improper catheter use, sexual activity, or cleaning. Additionally, hormonal fluctuations, urinary tract abnormalities, and a compromised immune system—particularly in postmenopausal women—are risk factors.

Additionally, certain lifestyle choices can heighten the risk of UTIs. A dearth of hydration, prolonged retention of urine, and the use of aggravating feminine hygiene products can foster an environment that is conducive to the proliferation of bacteria. Moreover, sexual activity has the potential to introduce microorganisms into the urethra, especially in females.

To reduce the risk of urinary tract infections, it is vital to adopt healthy practices. Adequate hydration facilitates the elimination of bacteria from the urinary tract, while adherence to proper sanitation practices, such as correct cleaning techniques, can avert bacterial re-introduction. Preventive measures include avoiding the use of abrasive products in the genital area and urinating before and following sexual activity.

Diagnosis And Symptoms Of Urinary Tract Infections

UTI symptoms must be identified to ensure prompt diagnosis and treatment. A strong, persistent urge to urinate, a searing sensation during urination, cloudy or pungent-smelling urine, and lower abdominal distress are typical symptoms. UTIs may occasionally result in fever and shivers, which may indicate a more serious infection that has progressed to the kidneys.

A medical professional will typically examine a urine sample for the presence of bacteria and white blood cells to diagnose a urinary tract infection (UTI). Further diagnostic evaluations, such as imaging studies or urine cultures, might be required in certain instances to ascertain the precise bacteria responsible for the infection and determine the degree of involvement.

Although antibiotics are the principal therapeutic approach for urinary tract infections (UTIs), lifestyle and dietary adjustments may serve as supplementary measures to medical interventions. Certain dietary components may aid in urinary tract health promotion and infection prevention.

1. Citrus and Cranberry Smoothie:

• Components:

• 1 cup unsweetened or fresh cranberry juice

• 1/2 cup Greek bland yogurt

Half a cup of citrus juice

• 1/2 cup berries, including blueberries and strawberries, chilled

• Honey, 1 teaspoonful (optional)

Instructions (•):

Whisk together every ingredient until uniform.

• Consistently consume this smoothie, as cranberries are recognized for their potential to inhibit bacterial adhesion to the walls of the urinary tract.

2. Roasted Salmon with Parsley and Garlic:

• Components:

Salmon fillets—2

• 2 minced garlic cloves

• 2 teaspoons minced fresh parsley

1) Tonne of olive oil

• Pepper and salt to flavor

Instructions (•):

• Preheat to 400°F (200°C) the oven.

• In a basin, combine garlic, parsley, olive oil, salt, and pepper.

• Bake the salmon fillets for 15 to 20 minutes after coating them with the mixture.

Garlic possesses antimicrobial properties, whereas parsley promotes urinary health by acting as a diuretic.

3. Salad of Vegetable Quinoa:

• Components:

• 1 cup quinoa, cooked

• 1 cup halved cherry tomatoes

One cucumber, chopped

• 1/2 cup sliced red bell pepper

• 1/4 cup grated feta cheese

(2) teaspoons of extra virgin olive oil

• 1 tablespoon vinegar balsamic

• Pepper and salt to flavor

Instructions (•):

• In a basin, combine the quinoa, tomatoes, cucumber, bell pepper, and feta.

• Whisk together olive oil, balsamic vinegar, salt, and pepper in a separate basin.

• Distribute the dressing over the salad while gently tossing.

• Quinoa is a fiber-rich whole grain, and the vegetables contribute vital nutrients that are integral to one's overall well-being.

Although these remedies cannot substitute for medical treatment, they can serve as beneficial supplements to a comprehensive strategy for preventing and managing urinary tract infections. For accurate diagnosis and treatment, it is critical to consult a healthcare professional; however, these recipes may serve as a supplement to prescribed medications and lifestyle modifications.

By incorporating a diet abundant in nutrients that promote urinary tract health, one may potentially decrease the occurrence of urinary tract infections (UTIs) and enhance overall health.

CHAPTER TWO

Recipes For Urinary Tract Infections (UTIS): An Organic Method For Prevention

Urinary tract infections (UTIs) are prevalent bacterial infections that predominantly impact the bladder and urethra, which comprise the urinary system. Although antibiotics and other medical interventions are essential for the treatment of urinary tract infections (UTIs), there is an increasing interest in preventive measures such as dietary adjustments. By including particular recipes in your daily regimen, you can support a comprehensive strategy for preventing urinary tract infections.

Preventive Measures

UTI prevention necessitates adherence to a cohesive regimen of dietary habits, hygiene practices, and lifestyle decisions. In addition to proper personal hygiene and adequate hydration, dietary modifications are crucial in the prevention of urinary tract infections (UTIs). The following are several crucial dietary strategies:

1. Enhanced Fluid Consumption: Sufficient hydration is an essential factor in the prevention of urinary tract infections. Water consumption aids in the elimination of microorganisms from the urinary tract, thereby decreasing the likelihood of infection. It is advisable to integrate water-rich fruits such as cucumber and watermelon, as well as medicinal beverages, into one's daily regimen.

2. Probiotic-Rich Foods: Probiotics, which are frequently termed "beneficial bacteria," support the maintenance of a harmonious microbiota in the gastrointestinal and urinary tracts. Kimchi, yogurt, kefir, and sauerkraut are all outstanding sources of probiotics. Consuming these can strengthen the body's innate defenses against urinary tract infections.

3. Restricting the Intake of Sugar and Caffeine: Overindulgence in sugar and caffeine may foster a

conducive environment for the proliferation of bacteria. By reducing your consumption of sugary beverages, chocolates, and caffeinated drinks, you can destroy microorganisms in the urinary tract.

4. A balanced diet, comprising a selection of fruits, vegetables, whole cereals, and lean proteins, is conducive to promoting holistic health, which encompasses the maintenance of a strong immune system. Foods abundant in essential nutrients furnish the body with the requisite resources to efficiently repel infections.

5. Garlic and onions are both botanical specimens that exhibit inherent antimicrobial characteristics. By incorporating these components into your recipes, you not only enhance the taste but also help to establish an environment that is less favorable for the proliferation of microorganisms.

The Criticality Of Hydration

Assuring adequate hydration is a straightforward and highly efficacious approach to UTI prevention. Water functions as an inherent urinary tract disinfectant, aiding in the elimination of pathogens and impeding their ability to adhere to the walls of the bladder. Importance of hydration in preventing urinary tract infections:

1. The concentration of microorganisms in the urine can be diluted through the consumption of sufficient water. This increases the difficulty of bacterial adhesion to the urinary tract and subsequent infection.

2. Consistent Urination: Adequate hydration facilitates frequent urination, a vital process for the removal of pathogens from the bladder. Prolonged retention of urine promotes bacterial proliferation, thereby augmenting the likelihood of infection.

3. Improved Immune Function: For optimal immune function, adequate hydration is vital. Maintaining

adequate hydration aids the immune system's endeavors to defend against infections, including those that affect the urinary tract.

4. Preventing Recurrences: Consistent hydration is a critical determinant in diminishing the probability of subsequent infections for individuals who are susceptible to recurrent urinary tract infections. It is a straightforward and readily available method for proactively improving urinary tract health.

Including adequate hydration in your daily regimen is an uncomplicated yet effective preventive action. Aim for a minimum of eight 8-ounce glasses of water daily, and alter your consumption according to climate and level of physical activity.

Cranberry And Urinary Tract Infections

Cranberry and urinary tract infection (UTI) associations have been the subject of research and discussion. Cranberry is frequently suggested as a natural UTI prevention remedy.

The preventive effect is thought to be primarily attributed to proanthocyanidins, which hinder bacterial adhesion to the walls of the urinary tract. Here's how cranberry can be incorporated into your strategy for preventing UTIs:

1. Cranberry Juice: Cranberry juice, when consumed unsweetened, may reduce the ability of microbes to adhere to the membrane of the urinary tract, thereby preventing UTIs. Notwithstanding this, it is critical to select an unadulterated, pure variety to circumvent the inclusion of added carbohydrates that may potentially worsen the issue.

2. Cranberry Supplements Cranberry capsules and other cranberry supplements are available for those who find it difficult to ingest cranberry juice regularly. These alternatives offer a concentrated form of the active compounds while excluding the added carbohydrates that are commonly found in commercial juices.

3. By integrating fresh or dried cranberries into one's preparations, an additional method of capitalizing on the potential UTI prevention benefits of cranberries can be achieved. Incorporate them into yogurt, smoothies, or salads for a flavorful and nutritious twist.

It is essential to note that although cranberry can be a beneficial addition to your UTI prevention regimen, it does not function as a remedy for active infections. Moreover, before increasing their cranberry consumption, individuals with a history of kidney stones should consult a healthcare professional.

Probiotics To Prevent UTIS

Probiotics are living microorganisms that, when ingested in sufficient quantities, bestow health advantages. Although frequently linked to digestive health, recent studies indicate that probiotics might also contribute to the prevention of urinary tract infections (UTIs) through the maintenance of a healthy microbial balance. The following describes how to include probiotics in your UTI prevention regimen:

1. Kefir and yogurt are examples of fermented dairy products that are abundant in probiotics. By including these in one's diet, a healthy balance of microbes in the gastrointestinal tract and, by extension, the urinary tract can be maintained.

2. Probiotic Supplements: Probiotic supplements provide a convenient method to increase your probiotic intake. They are available in a variety of forms, including capsules, granules, and chewable tablets. Consider purchasing dietary supplements that contain strains recognized for their potential urinary health benefits.

3. Fermented foods such as sauerkraut, kimchi, and miso, in addition to dairy products, have the potential to foster a varied and advantageous intestinal microbiota. Immune function is correlated with gastrointestinal health, which may have an indirect effect on urinary tract health.

4. Prebiotics: Supplementing probiotics with prebiotics in one's diet can further enhance their proliferation and functionality. Prebiotics, which are present in foods such as garlic, onions, scallions, and avocados, are nondigestible fibers. They function as a source of fuel for advantageous microorganisms.

Although probiotics exhibit potential in the prevention of urinary tract infections, individual responses may differ. It is recommended to incorporate probiotics into one's diet progressively and seek guidance from a healthcare professional before doing so, particularly if one has pre-existing health conditions.

In summary, UTI prevention necessitates a comprehensive strategy that surpasses the use of antibiotics. Individuals can promote urinary tract health through the incorporation of hydration, mindful dietary choices, and specific food items. Although these preventive measures may prove beneficial in managing urinary tract infections, those who experience symptoms or have a medical history of recurrent infections should seek the guidance and treatment of a healthcare professional. It is important to bear in mind that a comprehensive strategy for preventing urinary tract infections (UTIs) encompasses a blend of adjustments to one's lifestyle, adherence to proper sanitation protocols, and consumption of a balanced diet abundant in beneficial nutrients.

CHAPTER THREE

Components Of A UTI-Friendly Diet

A UTI-friendly diet should emphasize nutrients that strengthen the immune system and promote urinary health. The following nutrients, when incorporated, may help create an environment that is less favorable for the proliferation of bacteria:

1. Cranberries and blueberries, among others, are antioxidant-rich and contain compounds that may inhibit the adhesion of microbes to the walls of the urinary tract. Consuming these fruits can serve as a delectable means of enhancing urinary health.

2. Probiotics: Fermented foods abundant in probiotics, such as yogurt and kefir, can support the maintenance of a healthy bacterial equilibrium in the gastrointestinal and urinary tract. Maintaining this equilibrium is vital to avert the proliferation of detrimental bacteria that may result in urinary tract infections.

3. Garlic: Antimicrobial in nature, garlic potentially aids in the fight against microorganisms. Incorporating garlic into one's diet not only serves to augment flavor but also potentially confers advantages for urinary health.

4. Spinach and kale, among other dark leafy vegetables, are rich in folate and vitamin C, among other vitamins and minerals. These nutrients contribute to overall health and support the immune system.

5. Lean protein sources, such as poultry, fish, and tofu, should be prioritized. In addition to promoting immune function, protein is vital for a balanced diet; selecting lean options helps avoid consuming an excessive amount of saturated lipids.

6. Whole Grains: Fiber, which is found in whole grains such as quinoa and brown rice, is beneficial for digestive health. By preventing the accumulation of toxic substances in the body, a healthy digestive system can indirectly benefit urinary health.

7. Cucumber: Its high water content renders it hydrating and potentially aids in the elimination of pollutants. Maintaining adequate hydration is essential for maintaining urinary tract health and preventing urinary tract infections.

Caffeine-Friendly For UTIS

Effective hydration is vital for the prevention and treatment of UTIs. Incorporating specific beverages into one's daily regimen may potentially enhance urinary health.

1. Maintaining adequate hydration is among the most effective methods of UTI prevention. Water aids in the elimination of urinary tract microorganisms, thereby decreasing the likelihood of infection. Each day, consume a minimum of eight 8-ounce containers of water.

2. Cranberry Juice: Despite contradictory evidence, several studies indicate that cranberry juice may aid in preventing the recurrence of infections. Pure,

unadulterated cranberry juice is the best option for avoiding added sugar.

3. Herbal Teas: Specific herbal teas, including nettle tea and dandelion tea, contain diuretic constituents that may stimulate the production of urine. This enhanced urinary flow may facilitate the elimination of urinary tract bacteria.

4. Anti-inflammatory and antioxidant-rich, green tea possesses anti-inflammatory properties. Incorporating green tea into one's daily regimen potentially yields numerous health advantages, such as immune function support.

Recipes To Relieve Utis

By integrating UTI-friendly ingredients into delectable recipes, one can enhance the experience of following a supportive diet. Here is an easy recipe suggestion:

Salad Of Cranberry Chicken:

The following are the ingredients:

• Shredded grilled chicken breast

Mixed greens, including kale, arugula, and spinach

• Sliced strawberries and fresh blueberries

The shredded feta cheese

• Dried, dried cranberries

• Dressing of balsamic vinaigrette

Means of instruction:

1. Combine the dried cranberries, feta cheese, blueberries, strawberries, and mixed greens with the shredded chicken in a large basin.

2. Toss the salad gently to incorporate the balsamic vinaigrette dressing that has been drizzled over it.

3. Immediately serve as a revitalizing and UTI-friendly dish.

Supportive Herbal Teas For UTIS

In addition to providing solace and supplementary sustenance, herbal infusions may also have therapeutic properties. It is advisable to integrate the following herbal beverages into one's daily regimen:

1. Dandelion Tea: Dandelion tea may support kidney function and enhance urine production due to its diuretic properties. Incorporate a serving of dandelion tea into your daily regimen.

2. It is hypothesized that nettle tea possesses anti-inflammatory and urinary tract soothing properties. It can serve as a supportive and tranquil addition to your collection of botanical teas.

3. Chamomile tea is recognized for its potential to mitigate tension and induce a state of tranquility. Due to the potential influence of stress on immune function, the consumption of chamomile tea may indirectly promote urinary health.

4. Tea Made from Marshmallow Root It is believed that marshmallow root has a calming effect on the urinary tract. While additional research is required, marshmallow root tea has been reported to provide alleviation for urinary discomfort in some individuals.

In conclusion, beyond antibiotics, a holistic approach to managing UTIs entails additional measures. A diet conducive to urinary tract infections (UTIs) comprising appropriate foods, beverages, and herbal infusions may contribute to symptom prevention and relief.

A healthcare professional must be consulted, nevertheless, to ensure an accurate diagnosis and appropriate treatment. By adhering to a supportive diet and medical advice, individuals can proactively improve the health of their urinary tract and overall well-being.

Recipes For Urinary Tract Infections (UTIS): A Nutritious Approach To Wellbeing

Urinary tract infections (UTIs) are prevalent and frequently distressing ailments that impact a substantial global population, with a higher vulnerability among women compared to men.

Although medical intervention is essential for the treatment of urinary tract infections (UTIs), incorporating dietary decisions into a comprehensive self-care regimen can be beneficial in the management and prevention of these infections. In addition to being a nutritious and delectable addition to your routine, UTI-friendly recipes can also promote urinary health as a whole.

It is crucial, when preparing recipes for urinary tract infections, to prioritize ingredients recognized for their antibacterial and anti-inflammatory characteristics. The recipes ought to place an emphasis on maintaining adequate hydration, integrate foods that are rich in water, and incorporate ingredients that promote urinary system health. Consider the following nourishing and inventive UTI recipes:

1. Walnut and Cranberry Salad:

• **Components:**

Uncooked cranberries

Mixed greens, including kale, arugula, and spinach

Walnuts and walnuts

Feta cheese, a

• Dressing made with olive oil and balsamic vinegar

Cranberries are well-known for their antibacterial properties, which inhibit the adhesion of bacteria to the urinary tract wall and thus prevent UTIs. Incorporate them with feta cheese for a calcium boost and nutrient-dense greens, which are also abundant in omega-3 fatty acids and texture, respectively.

2. Salmon grilled with garlic and lemon:

• **Components:**

Salmon fillets (19)

Shoulder of garlic cloves

Lemon juice •

Olive oil •

Pungent dill

Garlic is renowned for its antibacterial properties, which render it a valuable component in recipes that are conducive to urinary tract infections. For a flavor explosion, combine garlic with salmon which is rich in omega-3 fatty acids, citrus, and fresh dill for added antioxidants.

3. Stir-fried quinoa and Vegetables:

• **Components:**

Quinoa, a

• Vegetable mixture (carrots, bell peppers, and broccoli)

Ginger and garlic

Soy sauce (2)

Sesame oil (11)

Quinoa is an exceptionally high-fiber and protein whole grain. This stir-fry, when combined with an assortment of vibrant vegetables and utilizing the antibacterial attributes of garlic and ginger, presents a delectable and urinary tract infection-friendly supper.

4. Yogurt Parfait in Greece:

• Components:

Greek yogurt •

• Blueberries and strawberries are berries.

Honey •

Perhaps almonds or muesli

Greek yogurt is an excellent source of probiotics, which help maintain a healthy balance of intestinal flora. Enliven the parfait with berries that are rich in antioxidants, drizzle with honey and garnish with crisp almonds or granola for a gratifying and urination-friendly treat.

In addition to highlighting ingredients that may possess anti-UTI properties, these recipes emphasize the importance of maintaining a balanced and nutritious diet.

Additionally, remember to consume plenty of water throughout the day to flush pathogens from the urinary tract, which is an essential function of adequate hydration.

CHAPTER FOUR

Ideas For UTI-Friendly Snacks: Indulge In Delights While Putting Urinary Health First

When coping with a urinary tract infection (UTI), snacking can be difficult because many common foods can worsen symptoms or impede the healing process. Nevertheless, one can indulge in delectable treats that not only gratify cravings but also promote urinary health with a little ingenuity. Consider the following UTI-friendly refreshment options:

1. Berry and Yogurt Smoothie:

• Components:

Greek yogurt •

• Strawberries and blackberries in a mixture

Bananas •

Honey •

Greek yogurt, berries, bananas, and a dash of honey are blended to create a silky and gratifying smoothie. Probiotics are present in Greek yogurt, whereas antioxidants and natural flavor are found in fruit.

2. Cups of cucumber and hummus:

• Components:

chop cucumbers

Hummus, a

Their-ripe tomatoes

Spend slices of cucumber to form miniature vessels, then stuff them with hummus. Complement with cherry tomatoes to create a crisp and reviving refreshment that is abundant in protein-rich hummus and hydrating cucumber.

3. Chia Seed and Almond Pudding:

• Components:

Almond milk •

Chia grains (Ci)

Vanilla extract, the

• Almonds, sliced

For a nourishing pudding, combine almond milk, chia seeds, and a trace amount of vanilla extract. Almond slices are used to garnish for added crunch and healthful lipids.

4. Whole Grain and Avocado Crackers:

• Components:

Avocado, a

Grain-containing crackers

Lemon juice •

Flaked red peppers

A squeeze of lemon juice and a pinch of red pepper flakes should be added to the mashed avocado. Consume this as a gratifying snack on whole grain crackers; it is an excellent source of fiber and healthy lipids.

These nibbles emphasize minimally processed, whole foods that promote urinary health. By incorporating such munchies into your regimen, you can manage UTI symptoms while maintaining a balanced diet.

Nutritional Supplements For The Prevention Of UTIS: Fortifying Your Defense

In addition to maintaining a balanced and healthful diet, nutritional supplements may also be utilized to aid in the prevention of urinary tract infections (UTIs).

Specific vitamins and minerals may reduce the risk of recurrent urinary tract infections (UTIs), support immune function, and foster urinary system health. Consider the following essential nutritional supplements to prevent UTIs:

1. Probiotics include:

Probiotic supplements comprise advantageous microorganisms that promote the maintenance of a harmonious intestinal microbiome. An association exists between a healthy gastrointestinal microbiome and a reduced likelihood of urinary tract infections. Consider probiotics that contain Lactobacillus or other similar strains; these may aid in preventing the proliferation of detrimental bacteria in the urinary tract.

2. C vitamins:

Vitamin C is renowned for its immunostimulatory attributes and its capacity to induce acidification in urine, thereby establishing an unfavorable milieu for bacterial proliferation. One should contemplate augmenting their consumption of vitamin C-rich foods, such as citrus fruits, strawberries, and bell peppers, or supplementing with vitamin C daily.

3. Cranberry dietary supplements:

Cranberry supplements, which are accessible in the form of pills or granules, offer a practical means of accessing the nutritional advantages of cranberries while avoiding excessive sugar intake. These dietary supplements potentially inhibit the adherence of microbes to the wall of the urinary tract.

4. Mannose D:

• It is believed that D-Mannose, a form of sugar, inhibits bacterial adhesion to the urinary tract membrane. It could prove to be especially beneficial for those who are susceptible to recurrent urinary tract infections. Supplements containing D-Mannose are offered in powder or capsule form.

5. Zinc:

Zinc is a vital mineral that contributes to the functioning of the immune system. Sufficient zinc levels have the potential to enhance the immune system, thereby decreasing the risk of bacterial infections. Zinc supplements may be contemplated in the event of inadequate dietary intake.

Before adding any supplements to your regimen, it is crucial to seek the advice of a qualified healthcare professional. They possess the ability to evaluate your specific requirements, identify possible drug interactions, and verify that you are administering the correct dosages.

CHAPTER FIVE

Changes In Lifestyle For The Management Of UTIS: Holistic Approaches To Health

Certain modifications to one's lifestyle, alongside dietary considerations and nutritional supplements, may aid in the prevention and management of urinary tract infections. By adopting these holistic approaches, one can reduce the risk of recurrent UTIs and promote overall health:

1. Remain Hydrated:

Sufficient hydration is an essential factor in the elimination of pathogens from the urinary tract. In addition to consuming water throughout the day, contemplate incorporating hydrating foods into your diet, such as watermelon, cucumber, and celery.

2. Maintain proper hygiene:

• It is critical to practice proper personal sanitation to prevent the transmission of bacteria. It is imperative to practice comprehensive genital hygiene by wiping from front to back and avoiding the use of harsh soaps or douches, which have the potential to disturb the delicate equilibrium of microorganisms.

3. Utilize breathable apparel:

• Select cotton undergarments that are breathable to reduce perspiration in the genital area and facilitate adequate ventilation. Pants that are too restrictive or made of synthetic materials should be avoided, as they can retain heat and moisture and provide a bacterial growth-promoting environment.

4. Urinate Consistently:

• Frequent bladder emptying aids in the elimination of pathogens. To mitigate the potential for bacterial contamination, it is advisable to excrete before and following sexual activity and to prevent prolonged urinary retention.

5. Exploration of Natural Remedies:

• Natural remedies, including essential oils (e.g., tea tree oil), herbal infusions (e.g., chamomile or dandelion), and heated compresses, have been reported to provide relief for UTI symptoms in some individuals. Nevertheless, it is imperative to seek the advice of a healthcare professional before attempting any alternative treatments.

6. Conquer Stress:

• Insufficiency of immune system strength due to chronic stress can increase the body's vulnerability to infections. Integrate stress-relieving practices, such as yoga, meditation, or deep-breathing exercises, into your daily regimen.

7. Consistently Engage in Exercise:

Consistent engagement in physical activity fosters optimal health, which includes the development of a robust immune system. Aim for a minimum of 150 minutes of exercise per week at a moderate intensity, such as cycling, leisurely strolling, or swimming.

A Healthcare Professional's Consultation

Although implementing lifestyle modifications, dietary modifications, snacking, and nutritional supplements can aid in the prevention of urinary tract infections (UTIs), it is imperative to seek the guidance of a healthcare professional to receive comprehensive treatment. Based on your medical history, a healthcare provider can evaluate the severity of the infection, prescribe the most suitable medications, and offer individualized guidance. Why it is essential to consult a healthcare professional regarding UTI treatment:

1. Precise Diagnosis:

• Symptoms of a urinary tract infection (UTI) may converge with those of other ailments, and self-diagnosis could result in unsuitable therapeutic interventions. A healthcare professional possesses the capability to conduct essential diagnostic procedures, including urinalysis, to precisely diagnose a urinary tract infection (UTI).

2. Prescription Pharmaceuticals:

• Antibiotics are frequently prescribed for the treatment of bacterial infections such as urinary tract infections. The appropriate antibiotic to prescribe is determined by the susceptibility of the bacteria causing the infection to various medications and the specific bacteria responsible for the infection.

3. Determination of Fundamental Causes:

• Recurrent urinary tract infections (UTIs) could potentially indicate the presence of underlying complications, including kidney stones, structural irregularities, or compromised immune function. A healthcare professional is capable of examining and treating these fundamental factor.

4. Continuation and Monitoring:

• By monitoring your progress throughout and following treatment, medical professionals can guarantee that the infection has been completely eradicated. Subsequent consultations provide the opportunity to modify the treatment regimen as necessary.

5. Preventive Measures:

A healthcare provider can provide individualized guidance regarding preventive measures, considering factors such as one's lifestyle, medical background, and preexisting conditions. This may encompass suggestions regarding adjustments to one's diet, level of hydration, and way of life.

6. Counseling and Education:

Healthcare personnel possess the ability to impart valuable knowledge regarding the prevention of urinary tract infections, proper sanitation practices, and modifications to one's lifestyle. Counseling sessions may encompass the exploration of concerns, inquiries, or affective dimensions about urinary tract infections (UTIs).

In summary, although incorporating UTI-friendly foods, recipes, and nutritional supplements into one's lifestyle can aid in the comprehensive management of urinary tract infections, it is crucial to retain the counsel of a healthcare professional. Precise diagnosis, suitable treatment, and continuous support for optimal urinary health are all guarantees of their expertise. Consult a medical professional immediately and without hesitation if you suspect a urinary tract infection (UTI) or experience recurrent symptoms; doing so is the most important and foundational measure in ensuring effective treatment and prevention.

Conclusion

In summary, the integration of particular dietary patterns can have a substantial impact on the prevention and management of urinary tract infections (UTIs). The aforementioned recipes, which are loaded with antibacterial and anti-inflammatory components, aid in the preservation of urinary system health.

Emphasizing hydration via cranberry-based beverages, herbal infusions, and infused water can aid in the elimination of microorganisms and promote urinary tract health as a whole. Moreover, by including probiotic-rich foods in one's diet, such as fermented vegetables and yogurt, urinary health can be indirectly influenced through the maintenance of a balanced gastrointestinal microbiome.

Incorporating ginger, turmeric, and garlic into recipes provides robust antibacterial and anti-inflammatory properties, which may aid in the prevention of urinary tract infections. In addition, a diet rich in fruits and vegetables supplies the body with vital antioxidants and vitamins, which strengthen the immune system in the face of pathogens.

It is imperative to emphasize that dietary modifications should not be regarded as a replacement for expert medical advice and treatment. It is advisable for individuals suffering from recurrent urinary tract infections (UTIs) to seek the advice of healthcare professionals to ascertain the root causes and formulate an all-encompassing course of treatment.

By incorporating these recipes that are suitable for urinary tract infections (UTIs) in conjunction with medical advice, one can essentially implement a comprehensive and preventative approach to urinary tract health.

THE END